Starve Your Cancer:

Intermittent fasting to starve your diseases and renew your metabolism.

J. Lawrence Tine

Table of contents

An analysis of the benefits and advantages of following a time-restricted eating protocol.

A look at the possible negative effects of following an intermittent fasting protocol. How real are these supposed dangers? And if possible, how may we mitigate some (or all) of these risks?

What is it?

A quick overview of some of the most recent and exciting research conducted regarding the possible metabolic origins for a host of modern diseases including cancer.

Interpretation of the findings of recent academic studies and what it may mean for us.

Chapter 7 - How to do intermittent fasting. *p 89*

A brief discussion of the various time restricted eating protocols as well as their respective pros, cons and methods of implementation.

Chapter 8 - Clarifications. p *101*

A chapter on how long you need to fast, what you may consume during a fast, what to eat when breaking a fast and what to eat for the greatest health and disease fighting benefits.

Foreword by the author

Good day Dear Reader

Thank you for purchasing this book.

It is with great joy that I present this information to you.

Cancer rates are increasing globally.

This includes increases in cancer rates in both the developed as well as in the developing world.

And although the brightest minds in the medical community are constantly at work trying to find new cures, solutions, and preventions for the diseases that plague the modern world, I think that it is good to occasionally take a step back and try and see the wood for the trees.

I think that it is no great overstatement to say that a lot of the modern diseases currently plaguing us is because of, or at least partly because of the food we are consuming.

Factory farming, herbicides, pesticides, fungicides and other poisons that are to be found on and in the foods we consume, as well as the depleted mineral content of the soil in which many of these foods are grown, together with the admission of growth hormones and low quality feeds to livestock have greatly changed the nature of the food that we consume.

There is also an over-abundance of cheap and easily obtainable calories because of the abundant and inexpensive supply of simple sugars.

These are sourced, from amongst others, cane sugar, beet sugar or high fructose corn syrup.

And whilst we should take a look at the effects of these foods on our metabolism, it is also worth noting that by simply allow our digestive system and metabolism time to react to these foods, that a lot of the negative effects that they cause in our bodies can be overcome, or at least diminished to a great extent.

This is where the theory and practice of time restricted eating comes into its own.

This is essentially what this book is about and what I am so excited to bring to you.

Like most modern people living in the world today I've had my fair share of health ailments and metabolic disruptions because of the modern foodstuffs and diet that we consume.

I've also been personally affected by cancer (although I have not had cancer myself) and I have seen firsthand the effects of making subtle dietary changes together with modern medicine can have on this dread disease.

Intermittent fasting and other protocols of time restricted eating seem to be gaining popularity and momentum in common parlance today.

And in an industry cluttered by fads, extreme diets and bad information I feel truly thankful that information such as this is beginning to see the light of day.

Intermittent fasting, although popular currently, is not a fad and is not unhealthy or harmful in any meaningful way.

In fact, what we now call intermittent fasting or time-restricted eating was for the greatest history of human beings on this planet simply called "eating".

An oversupply and overabundance of food was the exception and not the rule for the vast majority of human history.

As a result our digestive system likely developed to go for extended periods of time without food and is designed to run efficiently in this manner.

This is both my own, as well as other far more esteemed researchers' point of view.

Intermittent fasting or other protocols of time restricted eating holds great promise when used in conjunction with proper nutrition, as well as the elimination of bad foodstuffs to offset a lot of the diseases, metabolic and otherwise, that plague our modern existence.

The overabundance of food is not a negative thing per se, as it has allowed the world to be fed to a great extent.

This is not to suggest that hunger does not exist anywhere on the planet anymore.

But it must be noted that rates of hunger, malnutrition, and starvation has been greatly diminished across the world in recent decades.

However, these improved industrial farming methods that have allowed the world to be fed to a far greater degree, it is not a blessing that comes without a curse as well.

We are modern people living in a modern world, with modern foods, and with modern methods of producing those foods, and yet I believe that we should take a look at an ancient pattern of eating.

I believe we should develop and modernize this method of time restrictive eating to fit in with our modern lives, in order for us to enjoy the great abundance of the modern world, without succumbing to its diseases and its most extreme repercussions.

This book has been written with somber and sincere effort, referencing the latest research and studies conducted within the fields of nutrition, metabolic disease, and disease prevention.
It is with great joy that I present this book to you.

My hope is that you will find the information contained herein useful, practical and applicable.
Thank you very much for buying this book.

Best wishes and happy reading.

Lawrence

About this book:

This is a book containing research recently conducted by, amongst other institutions, the University of Southern California.

It contains research that is at the cutting edge of the intersection between nutrition and cancer research.

This book discusses a recently re-popularized theory known as the Metabolic Theory of Cancer.

The metabolic theory of cancer is not new, however.

New research and technology have simply brought this theory back to the forefront of cancer investigation.

This is a theory of cancer that is currently being researched by some of the top scientists and universities across the world.

This theory holds that nutrition and the foods that we consume have a far greater role to play in the creation of malignant tumors that have previously been thought possible.

Although this is currently still a theory, new and ongoing research has empowered some truly fascinating results regarding the effect of metabolism and digestion on the creation and growing of cancer cells.

This metabolic theory of cancer will be discussed in the pages of this book.

We will be looking at some of the studies that have been conducted recently, as well as the conclusions that these studies have reached.

We will also be looking at intermittent fasting as well as the role that it plays in the regulation of metabolic functions, as well as the implications that this research might have as an alternative way of combating cancer.

To be clear, this book does not seek to dissuade the reader from seeking professional conventional medical care.

It does, however, have as its aim the presentation of a non-harmful alternative that can be used in conjunction with conventional medical care in the fighting of cancer, as well as various other diseases.

In this book we will be looking at the following topics:

What is intermittent fasting?

In this chapter, we will discuss what intermittent fasting is and is not.

This book will also attempt to clear up a lot of the misconceptions regarding intermittent fasting, it will also attempt to explain the methods in which intermittent fasting works in our bodies.

With regards to our metabolism, the beneficial effects of intermittent fasting will be discussed at a later stage in the book.

The first section of the book is reserved for us to have a clear understanding of the foundations of intermittent fasting, in order for us to know what is meant when the term intermittent fasting is used.

The second section of this book will look at the benefits and advantages of intermittent fasting.

We will be explaining why the use of a restrictive time of eating has any bearing on our bodies and, with regards to our metabolism, we will see whether or not any benefits occur above and beyond simply the benefits that stem from fewer calories consumed.

This book will also take a look at the role that the sources of our caloric intake play in our overall health.

This is to say that there are three aspects of nutrition that needs discussion:

First of all, the amount of energy or calories consumed.

For a long time this was the only discussion tolerated within the medical establishment.

The theory can be broadly summarized as "calories in, calories out".

As new research is forthcoming, we in the nutrition field realize that the simple "calories in, calories out" theory is not conclusive.

New schools of thought within the field of nutrition then started espousing that, although the amount of calories matters significantly, that of equally great importance is the source of those calories.

This, of course, makes logical sense.

If a person obtains the roughly 2500 - 3000 calories per day that an adult human would on average require to maintain weight from doughnuts or from vegetables there would indeed be a difference in the health of the person.

Although person A, eating doughnuts for a total of 2500 calories per day, and person B, eating vegetables for a total of 2500 calories per day, both maintain their weight, I think that it is clear and logical to most readers that person B, the vegetable eater, will indeed be more healthy.

And so, for a relatively long while, ideas regarding nutrition have shifted to these first two theories.

Firstly, that the amount of calories consumed is all that matters.

Then secondly, and only much later on accepted as fact by the majority of the medical establishment, that the source of the consumed calories matters as well.

However, a third theory regarding metabolism and nutrition is now gaining traction.

This theory holds that, yes, the number of calories consumed matters, and yes, the source of the calories matters, but also that the timing of the consumption of the calories matters.

This is what the discussion of intermittent fasting later on in this book will we will be centered around.

We will be looking at the number of calories to be consumed roughly for men and women at various stages of life and activity levels.

We will also be looking at the preferred sources of the calories to be consumed.

However, the scope of this book is mainly concerned with the discussion of time restrictive eating patterns and the benefits that they hold for us. Both in terms of general health, as well as in combating various diseases, including most cancers.

The third section of this book will be looking at the possible dangers of intermittent fasting.

This book will take an objective view of time restricted eating patterns in order to ascertain whether or not the so-called dangers of fasting are real or not.

And if any danger that may arise from following a time restricted eating protocol does exist, this book will address the issue.

We will attempt to find ways of mitigating the possible negative effects of intermittent fasting, in order for us to reap the rewards of the positive effects and health benefits of intermittent periods of caloric restriction.

We will attempt to apply these mitigating factors to all of the current major patterns and protocols of time restricted eating.

The fourth section of this book will be looking briefly at the metabolic theory of cancer, what it entails, and why it makes logical sense.

We will also in this chapter be looking at new research conducted specifically to ascertain whether or not time restricted eating patterns, such as intermittent fasting, has any effect on cancer specifically.

This book will also discuss the various types of time restricted eating and intermittent fasting, as a number of varying protocols exist.

We will be discussing how to implement these various intermittent fasting protocols into the readers daily life, and we will also be discussing the pros and cons of each specific time-restricted eating protocol.

Lastly, this book will attempt to answer some of the most basic questions regarding intermittent fasting.

Questions such as what can be consumed during a fast, as well as for how long the fasting period should last.

This last section will also be discussing what foods to be consumed when breaking a fast, which foods to consume for general health, as well as which foods to consume for their general cancer-fighting properties.

I hope that you find great utility, insight, and knowledge from this book and that it will help to describe to you, and help familiarize you, the reader, with these exciting new developments in medical research, as well as clarify the potential implications for health, disease management, and disease-fighting that it holds.

The information provided herein is stated to be truthful and consistent, in that any liability, in terms of inattention or otherwise, by any usage or abuse of any policies, processes, or directions contained within is the solitary and utter responsibility of the recipient reader. Under no circumstances will any legal responsibility or blame be held against the publisher for any reparation, damages, or monetary loss due to the information herein, either directly or indirectly.

The author and/or the nom de plume of the author owns all copyrights not held by the publisher.

The information herein is offered for informational purposes solely and is universal as so. The presentation of the information is without a contract or any type of guarantee assurance.

The trademarks that are used are without any consent, and the publication of the trademark is without permission or backing by the trademark owner. All trademarks and brands within this book are for clarifying purposes only and are owned by the owners themselves, not affiliated with this document.

Chapter 1 - What is intermittent fasting?

In its simplest, most basic form intermittent fasting is simply periods of going without food (usually for periods of between 16 - 36 hours) followed by periods of eating.

The periods of going without food are obviously referred to as fasting.

Intermittent fasting in its most humble form is not a diet.

The periods of eating refers to eating normal, healthy food.

During the course of this book, some specific types of food will be encouraged for consumption during the eating window for maximum health benefits.

The reason being is that combining intermittent fasting with a healthy form of eating when breaking the fast allows us to basically double up on the benefits we get from following an intermittent fasting protocol.

The benefit of autophagy or cell renewal (as will be explained later on in this book) also increases in a fasted state.

Intermittent fasting also leads to increases in insulin sensitivity and increases in human growth hormone secretion.

It also allows for a little bit of a rest period for our digestive systems.

This rest period is as a result of the fasted portion of the intermittent fasting protocol.

For the maximum health benefit, we then combine this time restricted eating protocol with sensible and healthy foods that not only nourishes and restores us, but also protects us from various diseases.

Intermittent fasting is said to boost weight loss and this is becoming a more and more established fact as research continues to be conducted.

In many health and nutritional circles this knowledge is commonly known and accepted at the current time.

In fact, I'd be willing to bet that most practitioners of intermittent fasting do so for the weight loss and the fat loss benefits that intermittent fasting provides alone.

However, intermittent fasting provides us with numerous other, perhaps lesser-known health benefits as well.

Some of these additional benefits include improved cognition and mental health.

Additional benefits also include better brain health as well.

Furthermore, we can also expect better cardiovascular health as a result of following an intermittent fasting protocol, and crucially, as it relates to the scope of this book, intermittent fasting also gives us various digestive and metabolic health benefits.

These metabolic benefits relate to the disease-fighting properties of an intermittent fasting protocol.

Perhaps the most easily understood advantage from a digestive and metabolic health benefit standpoint is simply an extended period of rest for our digestive system, as well as lessened secretion of the accompanying hormones.

Reduced hormone secretion as a result of a period of not eating allows for a period of, amongst other hormones, no insulin secretion.

Although insulin has received a bad rap as of late, it is, in fact, a very important, very amazing hormone.

The problem is not insulin in and of itself, the problem is too much insulin.

Too much insulin is a result of consuming too many refined foods.

This is to say too many refined carbohydrates and empty sugars.

When consuming natural sugars, for example in the form of fruit, a good portion of natural fiber will be ingested along with the fruit.

The sugars and fiber are ingested together.

This fiber reduces the glycemic load or glycemic index of the fruit, allowing for slower absorption of the sugar in the fruit into the bloodstream, as well as a smaller amount of insulin having to be secreted.

As we will see in this book, the overabundance of insulin and it's a resultant metabolic disease, metabolic syndrome and type 2 diabetes causes many other negative health outcomes.

And, although the research is quite new, according to at least a couple of leading scientists and researchers the overabundance of insulin, as well as the resultant insulin resistance associated with it, can be linked to many different types of cancer.

This makes sense from a logical standpoint, as we will discuss.

Intermittent fasting allows for a period of not consuming any food and as a result the body receives a period of rest from digestion.

You see, digestion is a metabolically expensive function.

It is also a priority function.

Meaning that when you eat, the food ingested has to be digested.

However, if the body does not have to expend energy on digestion it can redirect energy to other bodily functions.

For example towards building up the immune system or repairing areas within our bodies where there is damage and accompanying inflammation.

The progressive, continuous, overwhelming ingestion of harmful substances, most likely in the form of improper food, is usually why we have chronic inflammation.

A period of not eating allows not only our digestive tract to rest, but allows the rest of our body to heal.

An amazing thing also happens when a fast is prolonged.

Because our bodies still have energy requirements, even if no ingestion is occurring.

And because the required energy still has to be obtained from somewhere, even when abstaining from calories for a long enough period, the body will start "eating itself".

Now, before you panic and think that this sounds like an absolutely horrible occurrence, please know that your body is designed much more intelligently then you would assume.

For you see, when your body starts cannibalizing itself, it does so through a process called Autophagy.

What happens during this process known as autophagy, a process during which your body starts to "eat itself", is that the body prioritizes for breakdown and cannibalization all the dying, suboptimal and not correctly functioning cells.

First, it cannibalizes these suboptimal cells as a means to produce energy for the body.

Autophagy does not target healthy cells for cannibalization initially.

Only in situations of an extreme fast, such as during a famine, will the body eventually start "eating", or cannibalizing healthy cells as well.

This will only occur in very extreme conditions of malnourishment because in such dire conditions the body will prioritize certain critical bodily functions over other, perhaps less important, bodily functions.

For example, during a famine muscle, which is a very metabolically expensive tissue, will be broken down for energy to keep the vital organs functioning.

This is why, when we see pictures of people having suffered a famine, their bodies are so incredibly worn out and malnourished.

Yet in many cases these people are still alive and, at least in the objective medical sense of the word, healthy.

This, of course, is not the point of intermittent fasting, as the damage done to by such a prolonged fast, where the body eventually begins consuming muscle mass, is very great.

Muscle mass is difficult to rebuild.

As a result, intermittent fasting does not go to those extremes.

It allows us to tap into the amazing power of autophagy, but just for long enough to recycle and consume our "not so great" cells, and not for so long as to start cannibalizing our healthy tissue.

As mentioned earlier, intermittent fasting is probably, and actually, a quite normal and healthy digestive protocol.

This is because intermittent fasting is probably closer to the way that our ancestors consumed food in the ancient past, and perhaps even up to the not so distant past.

But what about metabolism?

Won't my metabolism slow down?

Won't my body go into the famine mode?

And won't weight-loss become increasingly difficult?

Actually, no!

As this book will answer, later on, there is no need to be concerned about the metabolism slowing down.

As long as the calories consumed daily remains fairly consistent, and as long as daily consumption remains close to the number of calories consumed by the practitioner before embarking on an intermittent fasting protocol.

Of course, if weight loss is part of the objective of the time restricted eating protocol, then a slight reduction in daily calories can be maintained in order to facilitate it.

However, this level of caloric deficit will be only slightly lower than the maintenance level of calories required for a given period.

As a result, your body, thyroid, and metabolism will still receive the required signals that let them know that food is plentiful and readily available and that there is not a famine underway.

It might also be useful to, every now-and-then, not have an intermittent fasting day.

You might incorporate a non-fasting day as one day during a weekend, or maybe for a whole weekend, or perhaps for every second weekend or maybe for 5 days in a row during a month, etc.

There are various options that can be considered.

But, as a short answer, as long as the calories consumed during the eating window (meaning the period after the fast) remains broadly similar to the usual number of calories consumed by the practitioner during a normal, non-fasted day, then no ill effects on the metabolism have, as yet, been discovered by researchers.

It's important to remember that intermittent fasting is not a diet. It is simply a way of eating, and not-eating.

Certain people might practice intermittent fasting whilst also following a very low-calorie diet.

If metabolic slowdown occurs amongst these practitioners I believe that it would be very unfair to put the blame at the feet of intermittent fasting, and not at the feet of the restrictive low-calorie diet.

An intermittent fasting plan, properly followed and implemented, will allow the practitioner to consume lots and lots of fresh fruits and vegetables, as well as healthy animal products, if the practitioner is so inclined.

Daily metabolic and caloric needs will still be met.

Another question that some people might have is "why is intermittent fasting so popular currently?

"Is it just another weight loss a fad?"

The world of dieting and nutrition is notoriously full of fads.

We've seen low-fat diets, high-fat diets, low-carb diets, the Atkins diet, the Paleo diet, ketogenic diets, various forms of restrictive diets such as the grape diet, the prison diet, et cetera, et cetera.

On and on it goes...

Now, to be clear, some of the diets mentioned above are actually quite healthy and can be used as a blueprint for a way of eating for the rest of your life. (Low-carb, Ketogenic, Paleo, etc.)

And of course, some of the diets mentioned above are very unhealthy, restrictive and low caloric, with low levels of the nutrition required for optimum health.

Such diets will cause your body harm.

The problem is not the existence of so many different diets, the problem is the confusion that it causes.

So to answer the question "is intermittent fasting not just another diet fad?"

In all honesty, when gaging recent popularity, then, of course, intermittent fasting is a fad to a degree.

Or differently stated, the degree to which intermittent fasting has gained popularity at the current time may make it seem like a fad.

But this recent popularity is as a result of renewed interest, research, and analysis into this ancient way of eating.

But this way of eating (the intermittent fasting protocol) is not a diet, it is not about which foods to eat (although mention will be made in this book of some healthy food choices that should be incorporated into the feeding window of an intermittent fasting protocol, in order to read the maximum health benefits), it is about when to eat.

This book is primarily about giving an explanation of the hormonal and metabolic changes that periods without food produce in the body.

Thus, in short, yes, intermittent fasting is a fad because it is currently quite popular. A lot of people are interested in the subject.

But it is not a diet fad, as it is not a diet!

Intermittent fasting is just a modern phrase, our modern way of simply describing a way of eating that is quite ancient.

In all probability, for the majority of human existence what we now call intermittent fasting was simply the only way of eating.

I suspect that we wouldn't have to go back too far in the past to see what we call "intermittent fasting" or "time-restricted eating patterns" in the modern world was simply referred to as "eating" in an earlier time.

Intermittent fasting is natural and the human body is quite well adapted to go for slightly longer periods without food, without any ill effects, than a modern person would likely believe to be the case.

I do believe that it is fair to say that a lot of the diseases regarding nutrition in the past might have been diseases of lack of nutrition.

Today, especially in the western world however, the diseases of nutrition are diseases because of an overabundance of nutrition.

The problem is no longer "not enough food" - as it was for the vast majority of human existence.

Today the problem is too much food, and too much food of the wrong kind.

I'm not a purist. You will not go to hell for eating a doughnut.

I don't believe that a slice of pizza is a sin, but I believe that these types of bad foods should be treated in the same manner as any other vice.

There is a big difference between a person that smokes a cigar on New Year's Eve or on his or her birthday, and somebody that smokes a pack of cigarettes a day.

There is also a big difference between a person that has one low alcoholic beer after mowing the lawn, or perhaps a glass of wine with a Sunday lunch, and a person that has a bottle of vodka per day.

Similarly there is a massive difference between a person that has a slice of cake on his or her birthday, and maybe a pizza once a month during movie night at home, and the person that lives on processed junk foods for breakfast lunch and dinner day in and day out, week by week, month by month, year in and year out.

A lot of well-meaning health gurus will tell you to avoid these foods at all cost, and of course, they would be technically correct in doing so, because these foods are harmful.

However, I live in the real world and I imagine that you do too.

It is often said that perfection is the enemy of good enough.

Perhaps aiming for perfection is too large a goal to be an achievable target, causing a resultant failure and loss of motivation when it is not achieved.

Perhaps a better strategy is to stop aiming for perfection and start aiming for good enough.

This is far more achievable.

The only problem of "good enough" is that it is a question of balance.

And balance is a very individual parameter.

Meaning that each person must find his or her own balance.

Therein lies the difficulty.

Intermittent fasting and other forms of time restricted eating allows us at least some wiggle room so that we can focus on eating and consuming healthy foods (fruits, vegetables, organic healthy animal products) on a near constant basis.

Aiming for "good enough" also means that when we have a doughnut or a slice of pizza or a hamburger with a soda that we do not see it as a failure, or as an indication of some or other personal shortcoming.

Instead, we understand that perfection is for all practical reasons unachievable.

Make no mistake, some people get to be perfect in the diets they choose to follow.

But for most of us that is simply unrealistic.

Intermittent fasting allows us to live in the real world, to follow a healthy way of eating and not eating.

It is a practical protocol allowing the consumption of healthy foods when we eat, and to allow out or digestive systems enough time to rest and repair.

So that when we have the occasional slice of pizza or chocolate bar (and it is important that I stress occasional means occasional) it helps to minimize the negative effects of such foods.

Intermittent fasting is not a license to eat whatever you want when you are in your eating window, this must be very clearly stated.

Allowing for a fasted portion of each day simply allows us to mitigate the damage caused to our digestive systems and bodies in general when we do have a bite of chocolate.

As mentioned, these bad foods should be seen as just an occasional vice.

Just as there is a difference between a person that has a light beer on a Saturday after mowing the lawn vs a number of hard liquor alcoholic drinks daily.

And just as there is a difference between a person that smokes a cigar on his or her birthday or maybe on New Year's Day, versus a person that smokes a packet of Marlboros every day.

In exactly the manner explained earlier, there is a massive difference between a person that eats sugary cereal for breakfast, has a chocolate for an 11 o'clock snack, followed by a hamburger with fries and a soda for lunch, then scarfing down a packet of chips with a soft drink for an afternoon snack and then has pizza and beer for dinner, versus a person that remains in a fasted state each day, eats one or two nutritious meals each day and then has a slice of cake on his or her birthday.

Intermittent fasting will allow us to be more in tune with our digestive systems.

Following a time restricted eating protocol for a few days allows the cravings for the garbage we consume on a regular basis to dissipate and go away entirely in due time.

As mentioned intermittent fasting is a natural way of eating.

It is the way that our ancestors would have eaten for millennia.

The concept of "three square meals" a day is actually a modern invention.

We will see how we can use intermittent fasting instead as a more natural way of "eating, and then not eating" for maximum health benefits during the rest of this book.

But in summary intermittent fasting simply means the following: going for a period of time without any calories, in order for our digestive system to rest and repair, followed by healthy, nutritious eating squeezed into a smaller, designated "eating window".

Chapter 2 -Why use intermittent fasting?

Important note: The information contained in the following chapters is based on academic review studies and other peer-reviewed research. Academic papers may or may not be your idea of a fun, entertaining read. I certainly enjoy plowing through them. But I know that not every reader shares this opinion. Therefore, throughout this book I've included "further reading" sections including links to the original studies that the information in the chapter is based on. The purpose of this is twofold; first, it allows for an easy read to the reader that just wants to understand the basic benefits of intermittent fasting without needing to know the exact "how/why" it occurs, secondly, it allows the reader who wishes to dive in a bit deeper a way of doing so without interrupting the flow of the book. If you are reading a paperback you will just have to type the URL's provided into your favourite search engine. Sorry 'bout that - that's just the nature of paper. - Lawrence

An analysis of the benefits and advantages of following a time-restricted eating protocol.

At first glance to many people in our modern world, the entire concept of intermittent fasting might seem controversial, dangerous and perhaps slightly crazy.

However, as previously mentioned in this book, the modern way of eating ("three square meals per day") is, in fact, an invention of the modern world where industrial methods of agriculture have made an abundance of cheap sources of calories a reality.

It is in fact far more likely that a time restrictive eating protocol more accurately mimics the way that our ancient ancestors most likely consumed food.

In other words, long periods of no, or very few, calories combined with equally long periods of moderate physical exertion, punctuated by short periods of very intense physical exertion.

These periods of hunger and exertion would then be periodically alternated with periods of abundant food, rest, recovery, and merrymaking.

We can imagine members of some ancient tribe of hunters pursuing a large animal across rugged terrain for extended periods of time.

We can imagine these hunters then expending lots of energy when the final act of the hunt occurs, then dragging, carrying, butchering and preparing the food further uses energy.

A similar scenario can easily be imagined when foraging for roots or berries or seeds. Lots of moderate amounts of energy expenditure at a fasted, or at least calorie restricted state, followed by the consumption of food in a relatively short period of time.

We must also remember that modern methods of food preservation such as refrigeration are also modern inventions, therefore, although other methods of food preservation have existed for millennia, we can reasonably assume therefore that the hunted and gathered foods would have had to be consumed within a relatively short period of time.

Thus, it is entirely reasonable to assume that the human body has adapted, through long periods of time to be perfectly well suited, and perhaps even find as preferable a pattern of eating that involves slightly longer periods of going without food followed by periods of eating (or indeed feasting).

If we, therefore, assume that the pattern of eating that is mimicked by intermittent fasting is quite normal, and in certain conditions and applications even preferable to our modern "three square meals" pattern of eating, then we must therefore also assume that following a time restricted eating protocol will have certain beneficial aspects regarding our health.

The question then becomes twofold:

1. What are these benefits?
2. How do we apply a time restricted eating protocol to reap these benefits?

The second question will be addressed later on in this book.

But let us answer the first question, at least at a basic level.

It seems prudent at this juncture to mention that research with regards to intermittent fasting, time-restricted eating protocols, and their associated health benefits are ongoing and continuously being expanded on.

The benefits as presented here is current at the time of this writing.

If new research is uncovered and presented to the public this book will be updated and revised as required.

Having said all that, let's dive into some of the benefits of intermittent fasting:

Broadly speaking we can expect to experience greater levels of Human Growth Hormone (HGH) to be secreted, levels of insulin within our bloodstream to be reduced and the process of cell repair and restoration known as autophagy (more on this later in the book) to be increased.

Placing the body in a fasted state for a relatively short period of time will also, according to recent research, and contrary to popular belief, increase the metabolic rate, thus increasing the number calories burned during the day, even whilst at rest.

This is known as an increase in the Basal Metabolic Rate of a person.

A drop in blood sugar levels has as an added advantage a reduction in insulin resistance.

Lower blood sugar levels accompanied by reduced insulin resistance helps in the prevention of diabetes.

Placing the body in a fasted state also improves heart and cardiovascular health.

Furthermore, intermittent fasting facilitates the growth of nerve cells in the brain.

This might mean that regular intermittent fasting could potentially offer protection against degenerative brain conditions such as, for example, Alzheimer's disease.

Let us now look at some of these purported benefits in slightly more detail.

The benefit of intermittent fasting on weight loss and fat loss:

At the most basic level, following a time restricted eating protocol such as one of the various different intermittent fasting protocols to be discussed later on in this book will mean that fewer meals are consumed during the course of the day.

Provided that a person does not binge and eat massive amounts of calories during their eating window, said person will end up consuming fewer calories.

Consuming slightly fewer calories than is required for lean body mass management is perhaps the most effective way to lose weight and also lose body fat in a permanent way.

Very rapid fat loss due to a severe calorie restricted diet will place the body in a stressed state as well as disrupt the metabolism.

As soon as regular amounts of calories are consumed again the metabolism will kick into gear and induce hunger.

This type of hunger cannot easily be overcome by willpower as your body has been trained to believe that food is scarce and therefore induces you to consume large amounts of food whilst it is available.

Therefore a sensible way to lose weight and body fat permanently is to still consume relatively high amounts of calories, only slightly less than maintenance levels each day.

For most people, in general (and there, of course, is a significant range of fluctuation between individual persons) your daily maintenance calories could be reasonably be estimated by taking your lean body weight in pounds and multiplying it by 14 and by 17.

Your daily maintenance calories will be somewhere between those two values.

Age, activity level, exposure to extreme temperatures and individual differences will play a role in determining the exact number of calories required for weight maintenance.

What is meant by the term "lean body mass"?

Obviously, when a person is overweight we cannot use their total weight in pounds in order to determine daily maintenance calories.

Therefore we want to use a weight that is reflective of normal, healthy body fat levels to use in the aforementioned calculations.

The most accurate way to determine this number is to measure your body fat.

Methods of determining body fat such as calculating BMI through simple height x weight or height x waist measurement calculations are not endorsed as they are too simplistic, inaccurate and error-prone.

Various methods can be used to determine body fat level.

The most accurate method for determining body fat level in my estimation is by using body fat calipers.

Body fat calipers are basically a pair of pliers that is used to measure the amount of subcutaneous fat that a person carries and from this measurement calculate a fairly accurate estimate of total body fat levels.

These can be purchased at most health stores or pharmacies for a couple of Dollars and is well worth the investment.

Instructions on how to use the calipers will be included with the calipers.

Once your body fat has been calculated, compare it to the below;

For men, the normal, acceptable level of body fat is between 18-25%

For women, the normal, acceptable level of body fat is between 25-31%

Calculate your body fat using body fat calipers.

Subtract the amount of weight above the acceptable levels mentioned above.

This will give you your lean body weight.

Use this weight, in pounds, and multiply by 14 and 17.

Use these numbers as your lower and upper levels of calories to be consumed daily for healthy weight maintenance.

For example, a 220 pound male with 20% body fat (within the acceptable level) will have the following calculations:

220 x 14 = 3080 calories at the lower level.

220 x 17 = 3740 calories at the upper level.

If this same person weighs 220 pounds with 40% body fat (15% body fat above the acceptable level) the caloric maintenance calculations will be as follows:

220 x 0.15 (15% of body weight that is over the acceptable level of male body fat) = 33 pounds of excess fat.

220 - 33 = 187 lean body weight.

Then;

187 x 14 = 2618 calories at the lower level.

187 x 17 = 3179 calories at the upper level.

These calculations give us a range of daily caloric intake for healthy weight management.

For healthy, sustained weight loss that does not place the body in a stressed state where rebound weight gain is bound to happen when normal eating resumes the following rule should be observed;

Eat a diet that has a deficit of 500 calories per day or 3500 calories per week to lose approximately one pound of body fat.

Following an intermittent fasting protocol and eating fewer meals per day makes consuming a slight deficit of calories far easier as you will consume two (or perhaps only one, depending on the intermittent fasting protocol that you decide to follow) nutritious, fulfilling meals per day that will leave you feeling satiated.

Your body will grow accustomed to the periods of fasting. As a result, the hunger pangs that may occur during the fasting period will be manageable and not unpleasant in due course.

But apart from weight loss occurring due to fewer calories consumed, intermittent fasting also enhances hormonal function which helps to facilitate additional weight loss.

Lower levels of insulin, more human growth hormone and noradrenaline, caused by remaining in a fasted state for an extended period of time all increase the breakdown of body fat and using this fat as a source of fuel for the body.

Studies have shown short-term fasting (such as intermittent fasting) can increase metabolic rates by as much as 14%.

Further reading:

*https://www.ncbi.nlm.nih.gov/pubmed/240
5717*
*https://www.ncbi.nlm.nih.gov/pubmed/108
37292*

Thus intermittent fasting not only causes fewer calories "in" (by the practitioner eating fewer meals), it also causes more calories "out" (through elevated metabolism).

Still worried about your metabolism slowing down?

A recent review study shows that, when compared to extended caloric restriction, short term caloric restriction (intermittent fasting) causes less muscle loss.

Further reading:
*https://www.ncbi.nlm.nih.gov/pubmed/2141
0865*

A lower risk of type 2 diabetes

A 2014 review study published in the Translational Research Journal claims that intermittent or alternate day (a variation of a standard intermittent fasting protocol) fasting shows great potential for weight loss, lower blood glucose levels (blood sugar) and lower levels of insulin.

These factors combine to reduce the risk of type 2 diabetes.

Further reading:
https://www.sciencedirect.com/science/article/pii/S193152441400200X#bib24

Researchers have also found that in overweight and obese adults there exists lower levels of insulin sensitivity.

This is a marker for type 2 diabetes.

Intermittent fasting has been shown to increase insulin sensitivity, thereby reducing the risk of type 2 diabetes.

Improved heart health.

A study from 2016 shows that a time restricted eating protocol can lead to a slower heart rate, lower blood pressure, reduced bad cholesterol and fewer triglycerides.

Triglycerides are a type of fat found in the blood.

Triglycerides are positively correlated to increased risk of heart disease.

Further reading:

https://www.ncbi.nlm.nih.gov/pmc/articles/ PMC5411330/
https://www.medicalnewstoday.com/article s/9152.php
https://www.medicalnewstoday.com/article s/237191.php

Improved brain health

In various animal studies, researchers have also found that intermittent fasting shows a decreased risk of various neurological disorders.

Some of these disorders include, amongst others, Parkinson's disease, stroke, and Alzheimer's disease.

Further reading:
https://www.ncbi.nlm.nih.gov/pmc/articles/ PMC5411330/
https://www.medicalnewstoday.com/article s/159442.php
https://www.medicalnewstoday.com/article s/323396.php
https://www.medicalnewstoday.com/article s/7624.php

A reduced risk of cancer

In recent studies, it has been discovered that time restricted diets such as a sensible intermittent fasting protocol could delay the onset of tumors.

It is important to note that these results were obtained from animal studies.

It nonetheless shows great promise for using intermittent fasting as a way to supplement traditional cancer treatments

Obesity has also been shown to be a risk factor in various types of cancer.

Intermittent fasting and a return to healthier levels of body fat could help to, therefore, reduce the risk of many different forms of cancer.

More on obesity, metabolism, and cancer here:
https://www.ncbi.nlm.nih.gov/pmc/articles/PMC5411330/
https://www.ncbi.nlm.nih.gov/pmc/articles/PMC5411330/

Chapter 3 - Possible dangers of intermittent fasting.

A look at the possible negative effects of following an intermittent fasting protocol. How real are these supposed dangers, and if possible, how may we mitigate some (or all) of these risks?

Risks of Intermittent Fasting

Many people are concerned that following a restrictive eating protocol will lead to unhealthy eating patterns.

This raises the specter of eating disorders.

Will intermittent fasting cause eating disorders?

This fear is largely unfounded as the goal of intermittent fasting is not caloric restriction.

The goal is to simply consume our daily calories in a shorter eating window.

A slight risk of binge eating might exist during the first few days of starting an intermittent fasting protocol.

This is simply because for most of us this will be the first time in our lives that we willingly chose to forego regular eating.

We might initially simply be hungry.

In our modern world, we are trained to fear hunger.

We come to experience it as unpleasant.

When in fact it is quite a normal thing.

Within a few days the hunger will transform into a surprisingly pleasant feeling.
It will lessen.

It won't be very severe.

In fact, it will become quite mild, in many cases unnoticeable.

Once this happens the possibility of binge eating at the end of a day will cease to be a factor.

Binging on bad foods during the eating window will erase many of the positive benefits of intermittent fasting.

Therefore it must not become a pattern.

Attempt to eat healthy meals at the end of the fasted period as soon as possible.

But there is no great risk inherent in intermittent fasting.

Metabolic disruptions are caused by malnutrition, not by time restricted fasting followed by nutritious meals.

Various studies have shown that a sensible intermittent fasting protocol is safe and even beneficial.

Prolonged fasting (longer than 36 hours) can under certain conditions (such as with cancer patients) be detrimental.

Therefore the practitioner must ensure adequate, healthy food consumption during the eating window.

If this simple rule is adhered to then there is no great risk or negative effect in following an intermittent fasting protocol.

You will also not trigger a famine response in your body.

You will not lose muscle mass.

You won't lose all those gains that you so dutifully fought for in the gym.

In order to go into the famine state, you would have to be severely calorie restricted for a much longer period of time than a regular intermittent fasting fasted window allows for.

The famine response is triggered, you know, during an actual famine.

As long as you eat enough and eat sensibly during your eating window there are no negative effects suffered by following an intermittent fasting protocol.

Chapter 4 - The metabolic theory of cancer.

What is the metabolic theory of cancer?

Firstly, it is important to note that the metabolic theory of cancer is just that: a theory.

It stands in contrast to the genetic theory of cancer.

The genetic theory of cancer is the prevailing cancer theory today.

The genetic theory sees genetic malfunctioning and certain genetic predispositions as the fundamental cause of cancer.

However, the metabolic cancer theory was for a long time the preferred theory regarding the origins of cancer.

It is a well-researched theory.

A number of studies, stretching back nearly a century have shown evidence of its existence.
I hold a different view, however.

I believe that BOTH theories are in fact correct.

At least at their most basic, theoretical level.

I further believe that the metabolic theory holds primacy as an explanation for many cancers. What do I mean by "primacy"?

I believe that the improper control of our metabolism (eating lots of junk, for example) creates the optimal environment within our bodies for cancer cells to develop and grow.

This, of course, is not necessarily true of all cancers.

But I believe that a bad diet with a sedentary lifestyle and the host of other negative health activities in our modern world creates the perfect state for cancer to develop.

The genetic theory then comes into play by helping to predict exactly what type of cancer we would be most likely to develop - based on our genetic predisposition.

The main problem that I have with the genetic theory of cancer is that it seems fatalistic and predeterminist.

I do not believe that this is a view people should have.

In fact, if we understand that we can do a couple of simple things in order to greatly diminish the probability of cancer forming within our lifetimes then we would be much more likely to do those things.

The basic premise of the metabolic theory is that cancer cells consume more glucose and produce more lactate than normal cells.

This different cell metabolism is called the Warburg effect.

It is also known as aerobic glycolysis.

The Warburg effect has been observed and recorded in thousands of research studies.

This observance of aerobic glycolysis has lead to the development of treatment protocols that attempt to stop tumor growth.

These protocols attempt to achieve this by starving cancer cells of the glucose that they require in order to grow and survive.

Who was Warburg?

Otto Heinrich Warburg, born 8 October 1883, died 1 August 1970, was a German medical doctor.

Warburg received the Nobel prize in physiology or medicine in 1931 for "the discovery of the nature and modes of action of the respiratory enzyme".

Dr. Warburg was also nominated for the Nobel prize 47 times over the course of his career.

With regards to aerobic glycolysis, let's first see how a normal cell functions:

In a normal cell, the mitochondria (the "engine" of the cell) uses a process of oxidative phosphorylation to create the energy the cell requires.

During this process, the cell gets its energy through respiration (aerobic).

Aerobic respiration tells us that it is a process that occurs in the presence of oxygen.

This type of respiration also needs glucose as fuel. The glucose gets burned for energy.

If respiration occurs in the absence of oxygen we refer to it as 'anaerobic respiration'.

This process is also known as fermentation.

Anaerobic respiration is not an efficient way to produce energy in normal cells.

Cells switch over to this method of respiration usually when the energy required is greater than the amount of oxygen and glucose available for energy production.

This is what happens when you have a beast training session in the gym.

It's also why your body is stiff and sore the next day. Because anaerobic respiration produces lactic acid.

In 1927 Dr. Warburg found that cancer cells, unlike normal cells, don't seem to need oxygen for energy.

He found that cancer cells tended to use glycolysis for energy. This occurred even when oxygen was available.

It became apparent to Dr. Warburg that cancer cells had found a way to produce required energy unrestricted by the inherent inefficiency of glycolysis.

The basic idea behind his theory is that if a cell gets some kind of damage to its mitochondrial function (damage to the cell's "engine"), that it will try to adapt by increasing glycolysis.

If it does succeed it will grow.
If it doesn't it will die.

Dr. Warburg believed that cancer cells were cells that had survived some type of mitochondrial damage as well as managed to adapt to using aerobic glycolysis as an energy production method.

The metabolic cancer theory was originally popular.

In the 1970s the genetic theory gained supremacism.

However, in recent years Dr. Warburg's theory has regained a lot of interest again.

This is because of modern technology and new research.

Recently it was found that:

Almost all tumors use aerobic glycolysis.

Furthermore, in 24 types of cancer, a general feature that has been noted is the over-expression of genes using glycolysis for energy.

This represents more than 70% of human cancers.

In recent years a slight modification of Dr. Warburg's original theory has been suggested.

The modified theory suggests that although many tumors may, in fact, have properly functioning mitochondria, that pockets of the tumor cells will have improper mitochondrial function caused by mutated genes.

These tumor cells are dependent on glycolysis for energy.

Research has suggested that tumor cells' mitochondria undergo "uncoupling" rather than permanent damage.

This is known as the mitochondrial uncoupling hypothesis.

Basically, it states that mitochondria in cancer cells can also undergo a metabolic shift and start using non-glucose sources of fuel for energy.

This hypothesis ties up some of the unexplained factors in the Warburg hypothesis.

It purports that tumor cells are somewhat metabolically flexible.

Thus tumors can adapt to different metabolic methods as they grow.

However, not all cancer cells undergo metabolic reprogramming.

Meaning that there seems to be some convincing evidence for the Warburg hypothesis in at least 70% of human cancers.

But that it may not be a cure-all, as some cancer cells can adapt their metabolism.

Therefore Intermittent fasting and a low carbohydrate diet can be very beneficial in starving cancer cells of the fuel they require.

But these approaches (intermittent fasting used in conjunction with a low carbohydrate eating plan) should be used in conjunction with modern, traditional oncology (chemotherapy and radiation).

As shown in research, intermittent fasting supports the effectiveness of chemotherapy.

Intermittent fasting also supports the immune system, therefore somewhat minimizing the detrimental effects of chemotherapy on the body.

Intermittent fasting should be seen and used as an aid in combating cancer.

Further reading:
Warburg, O. "KP, and E. Negelein." On the Metabolism of Cancer Cells (1924): 319-344.

Warburg, Otto. "On the origin of cancer cells." Science 123.3191 (1956): 309-314. http://mosao2.org/Article%20-%20Medicine/cancer_Otto_Warburg_oo.pdf

Seyfried, Thomas N., and Laura M. Shelton. "Cancer as a metabolic disease." Nutr Metab (Lond) 7.7 (2010): 269-70. http://www.nutritionandmetabolism.com/content/7/1/7

Koppenol, Willem H., Patricia L. Bounds, and Chi V. Dang. "Otto Warburg's contributions to current concepts of cancer metabolism." Nature Reviews Cancer 11.5 (2011): 325-337. http://fulltext.calis.edu.cn/nature/nrc/11/5/nrc3038.pdf

Cross, Carroll E., et al. "Oxygen radicals and human disease." Annals of internal medicine 107.4 (1987): 526-545.

Ames, Bruce N., Mark K. Shigenaga, and Tory M. Hagen. "Oxidants, antioxidants, and the degenerative diseases of aging." Proceedings of the National Academy of Sciences 90.17 (1993): 7915-7922. Page on pnas.org

Gutenberg, B. and, and K. O. Greenwich. "Genes of glycolysis are ubiquitously overexpressed in 24 cancer classes." Genomics 84.6 (2004): 1014-1020. Page on medicinabiomolecular.com.br

Gogvadze, Vladimir, Boris Zhivotovsky, and Sten Orrenius. "The Warburg effect and mitochondrial stability in cancer cells." Molecular aspects of medicine 31.1 (2010): 60-74.

Guo, Jessie Yanxiang, et al. "Activated Ras requires autophagy to maintain oxidative metabolism and tumorigenesis." Genes & development 25.5 (2011): 460-470.
http://genesdev.cshlp.org/content/25/5/460.full.pdf+html

Kaelin, William G. "SDH5 mutations and familial paragliding: somewhere Warburg is smiling." Cancer cell 16.3 (2009): 180-182.

WEINHOUSE, SIDNEY, et al. "On respiratory impairment in cancer cells." Science 124.3215 (1956): 267-272.

Wallace, Douglas C. "A mitochondrial paradigm of metabolic and degenerative diseases, aging, and cancer: a dawn for evolutionary medicine." Annual review of genetics 39 (2005): 359.
http://people.musc.edu/~rosenzsa/Spyropoulos/MitoMetabonAging.pdf

Yang, Ming, Tomoyoshi Soga, and Patrick J. Pollard. "Oncometabolites: linking altered metabolism with cancer." The Journal of clinical investigation123.9 (2013): 3652. http://www.research.ed.ac.uk/portal/files/15134728/Oncometabolites_linking_altered_metabolism_with_cancer.pdf

Mullen, Andrew R., et al. "Reductive carboxylation supports growth in tumor cells with defective mitochondria." Nature 481.7381 (2012): 385-388. http://basicmed.med.ncku.edu.tw/public/project/1166-1334226937-1.pdf

Guzy, Robert D., et al. "Loss of the SdhB, but Not the SdhA, a subunit of complex II triggers reactive oxygen species-dependent hypoxia-inducible factor activation and tumorigenesis." Molecular and cellular biology 28.2 (2008): 718-731. http://mcb.asm.org/content/28/2/718.full.pdf+html

Petros, John A., et al. "mtDNA mutations increase tumorigenicity in prostate cancer." Proceedings of the National Academy of Sciences of the United States of America 102.3 (2005): 719-724. http://www.pnas.org/content/102/3/719.full.pdf?sid=eaafccd5-c462-4ea6-89ca-6e7cc820de98

Ishikawa, Kaori, et al. "ROS-generating mitochondrial DNA mutations can regulate tumor cell metastasis." Science 320.5876 (2008): 661-664; Porporato, Paolo E., et al. "A mitochondrial switch promotes tumor metastasis." Cell reports 8.3 (2014): 754-766. http://ac.els-cdn.com/S2211124714005270/1-s2.0-S2211124714005270-main.pdf?_tid=070b7fac-5fcb-11e5-8cf1-00000aacb35d&acdnat=1442776310_923bcb28988921e2a2c0c500caeef50e

Lynne, Fe odor. "Die Rolle der Phosphorescence be Dehydrierungsvorgaengen und ihre biologische Bedeutung." Naturwissenschaften 30.25 (1942): 398-406.
(German language)

Samudio, Ismael, Michael Fiegl, and Michael Andreeff. "Mitochondrial uncoupling and the Warburg effect: molecular basis for the reprogramming of cancer cell metabolism." Cancer Research 69.6 (2009): 2163-2166.
http://cancerres.aacrjournals.org/content/69/6/2163.full.pdf+html

Derdak, Zoltan, et al. "The mitochondrial uncoupling protein-2 promotes chemoresistance in cancer cells." Cancer Research 68.8 (2008): 2813-2819.
http://cancerres.aacrjournals.org/content/68/8/2813.full.pdf+html

Amoedo, Nivea Dias, Mariana Figueiredo Rodrigues, and Franklin David Rumjanek. "MITOCHONDRIA: Are mitochondria accessory to metastasis?." The international journal of biochemistry & cell biology 51 (2014): 53-57.

MENENDEZ, JAVIER, et al. "The Warburg effect version 2.0: metabolic reprogramming of cancer stem cells." Cell Cycle 12.8 (2013): 1166-1179. http://www.tandfonline.com/doi/pdf/10.4161/cc.24479

Viale, Andrea, Denise Corti, and Giulio F. Draetta. "Tumors and Mitochondrial Respiration: A Neglected Connection." Cancer research (2015).

Frezza, Christian. "The role of mitochondria in the oncogenic signal transduction." The international journal of biochemistry & cell biology 48 (2014): 11-17.

Chapter 5 - Research and findings.

A quick overview of some of the most recent and exciting research conducted regarding the possible metabolic origins for a host of modern diseases including cancer.

A recent rodent study conducted by researchers at the University of Southern California found that mice receiving chemotherapy, whilst also going on an intermittent fasting protocol had a better immune system function.

Their immune systems were able to more effectively target and kill breast and skin cancer cells.
The rodents in the study, when in a fasted state, also produced more B cells and T cells (active killer immune cells) that destroy tumor cells.

Researchers also found that T regulatory cell, cells which in normal conditions give protection to tumors, where kept out of the tumors when the rodents engaged an intermittent fasting eating pattern.

It is also believed that the decrease of T regulatory cells within the tumors may have contributed to chemotherapy working better.

The same researchers also did a study to see if intermittent fasting protocols were safe to use with chemotherapy.

The study produced the following results;

Water only 48-hour fasts, and,

Restricted calorie diets that mimic fasting (conducted under medical supervision) were considered safe.

These findings show that intermittent fasting diets are safe to use in conjunction with chemotherapy.

These studies also show that fasting or an intermittent fasting diet along with traditional oncological chemotherapy treatment may be effective in slowing down tumor growth.

Study found here:
https://news.usc.edu/103972/fasting-like-diet-turns-the-immune-system-against-cancer/

For further research, also please see below:
Additional above-referenced study was published on July 11th, 2016 in the journal Cancer Cell.

Different studies have also looked at the effect of intermittent fasting on cancer survivors.

In one such study survivors of breast cancer engaged in 13 hour daily fasts.

The study showed a 36% reduction in cancer recurrence.

Longer fasting hours (15 hours in the case of this study) had a further increase in benefits.

Study details here:
https://jamanetwork.com/journals/jamaonc ology/fullarticle/2506710

Different rodent studies also show that 16-hour fasts, stretching over the rodents sleeping time, and having the rodents placed on a high-fat diet had better protection against abnormal inflammation, weight gain, and abnormal glucose metabolism, which are all factors that are associated with negative cancer outcomes.

Rodent studies obtained from the following research:
Hatori M, Vollmers C, Zarrinpar A, et al. Time-restricted feeding without reducing caloric intake prevents metabolic diseases in mice fed a high-fat diet. Cell Metab. 2012;15(6):848-860.

Chaix A, Zarrinpar A, Miu P, Panda S. Time-restricted feeding is a preventative and therapeutic intervention against diverse nutritional challenges. Cell Metab. 2014;20(6):991-1005.

Cancer seems to cause confusion in the patient's' immune system.

The immune system seems to become unable to find and destroy abnormal or damaged cells (such as cancer).

Research suggests that simply fasting periodically could trigger the immune system to seek and destroy these damaged cells.

It's important to note that cancer cells have their own protective cells.

These tumor protecting cells are known as T regulatory cells.

Studies have found that fasting has a great effect on the expulsion of these T regulatory cells.

Thus enabling the immune system to much more effectively target and fight the cancer cells.

Researchers hypothesize that the reduced ability of cancer cells to fight back against the immune system is because fasting causes the weakening of an enzyme known as HO-1 (heme oxygenase) inside the mitochondria of the T regulatory cell.

Cellular research on tumors has found HO-1 levels to be elevated in tumor cells.

HO-1 tricks the immune system into thinking that cancer cells are not bad. And that they, therefore, should not be killed.

Once the HO-1 is removed it is as if the immune system wakes up and says "hang on a minute, what are all these bad cells doing here? They must be destroyed!"

Fasting, or using a fasting mimicking diet such as regular intermittent fasting allows the body to identify and kill bad cells, whilst protecting the good cells.

Fasting also induces a process known as autophagy.

This is a process where, once the energy derived from food is depleted in the cell, the cell needs to find alternative sources of energy.

It does so by engaging in autophagy.

Autophagy literally means "self-eating".

But it's not as bad as it sounds.

During this fasted, depleted state your body starts to look at what's available inside the body itself for fuel.

It identifies all the sub-optimal, broken, dead, malfunctioning and diseased material within the body.

It then proceeds to "eat" these not-so-good materials, in order to obtain the energy and the building blocks required for the production of new, undamaged biological material.

Your body is very clever.

It doesn't cannibalize itself inefficiently.

As a result, during a short to medium term fast your body will only target, eat and reuse/remake what is required from sub-optimal biological material.

You can easily see therefore how fasting can be used in order for our bodies to preemptively get rid of any material which might cause problems in the future.

This includes eating the cells that may become (or may already have become) cancerous.

We conclude therefore that fasting helps us fight cancer because:

It starves cancer cells of the fuel it needs, at least to a degree (Dr. Warburg's hypothesis).

It removes HO-1 in order for our immune systems to not be hoodwinked anymore and thus attack the bad cells.

It allows autophagy to be induced, so our cells "eat" and discard all broken and damaged materials, whilst producing new cellular material to replace the "eaten" material.

It allows energy that would have otherwise been required for digestion to be used by the immune system for disease fighting.

Chapter 6 - Conclusions.

Interpretation of the findings of recent academic studies and what it may mean for us.

When taking into account the previous chapters we can conclude that:

For people with various types of cancer, that intermittent fasting holds a number of benefits.

Research shows that fasting, including intermittent fasting, can slow down tumor growth.

Fasting has also been shown to reduce the detrimental side effects of traditional oncological treatments (such as chemotherapy).

Studies have also shown an increase in survival rates in patients.

Intermittent fasting has also been shown to enhance and increase the effectiveness of the immune system.

Overall, and although research is still ongoing, intermittent fasting has been shown to be of benefit to cancer patients when used in conjunction with traditional cancer therapies.

One of the negative effects of chemotherapy is that it suppresses the immune system.

This, of course, is not a good thing, as we would like our immune system to join the fight against the cancer cells.

Intermittent fasting has been shown to raise the levels of bone marrow within practitioners.

Bone marrow is where the fighting cells of the immune system are created.

These include T-cells and B-cells that target tumors.

Elevated bone marrow levels due to intermittent fasting have even been observed in patients using chemotherapy medication.

Fasting also induces autophagy, which as previously mentioned, triggers the body to destroy ("eat") all the old, broken cells within the body.

Autophagy recycles this damaged material for primarily energy production.

Autophagy has effects greater than only cancer-fighting.

Autophagy also combats viral infections and parasites.

Autophagy, and fasting in general, also starves cancer cells by stopping the availability of the nutrients required by cancer cells to survive and grow.

This can lead to a slow down and perhaps even a decrease in the growth of tumors.

For more, see here:
https://www.naturalhealth365.com/fasting-cancer-cells-2238.html

Think of it this way:

The amount of energy available within the body is not infinite.

This is why we have to eat.

The energy obtained from food enables the body to perform a number of needed bodily functions.

These include, amongst others, movement, immune system antibody production, brain function, breathing and respiration, the pumping of blood throughout the body, digestion, new cellular growth, etc.

All of these functions require energy.

Some of these are more metabolically expensive than others.

This means that some bodily functions require more energy in order to function correctly.

Digestion in particular requires lots of energy.

Digestion also requires large quantities of blood in order to operate efficiently.

This means that digestion diverts energy away from other bodily functions where it may also have been required.

Furthermore, because food will contain outside pathogens (not necessarily a bad thing), eating will increase the load on the immune system.

Eating will cause an increase in immune activity.

Thus by fasting (i.e. NOT eating), we can experience a decrease in inflammation.

Because an elevation in immune activity will lead to more inflammation.

Please note, eating itself is not bad.

It is obviously necessary for survival.

However "what" we eat can significantly elevate or decrease the amount of immune activity triggered by the ingestion of food and its accompanying pathogens.

Remember also that if we prolong the period without food yet still ingest our required calories during our eating window, that we will have the best of both worlds.

We will not become malnourished. Remembering that our immune system and other bodily functions do require energy.

Yet, we will reap all of the benefits that fasting provides. Including a reduced immune response and accompanying inflammation that is triggered by eating.

Fasting decreases the release of IGF-1, a growth factor that has been linked to aging, tumor progression and increased risk of cancer.

Okay, but when we then do eat, what should we eat?

Well, research conducted during the last number of years suggests that a low carbohydrate approach seems to be most beneficial for cancer-fighting.

This applies in a direct way, i.e starving the cancer cells of the "food" they need to grow.

But it also applies in an indirect way.

Low carbohydrate eating has shown a significant decrease in the development of metabolic diseases such as metabolic syndrome for example.

These metabolic diseases have also been shown to have a positive correlation with the development of cancer.

Diets high in refined carbohydrate increases the secretion of IGF-1.

IGF-1 is an insulin-like growth factor.

As stated earlier, IGF-1 is linked with aging and tumor growth.

Thus a diet devoid of refined carbs inhibits the levels of IGF-1 and its resultant negative metabolic effects.

Concluding the conclusions:

Intermittent fasting has a number of beneficial properties that lower cancer risk, helps the body fight cancer cells by starving the cancer cells themselves whilst removing their disguise from the immune system.

Fasting also boosts the immune system. It also allows for more energy to be diverted to immune activity when the body is not preoccupied with digestion.

Bone marrow is increased, this means that the negative effects of chemotherapy are lessened to a degree.

Autophagy is induced causing the bad biological material to be "eaten" by the body.

IGF-1 insulin-like growth factor is diminished. IGF-1 has been linked to aging and tumor growth.

Chapter 7 - How to do intermittent fasting.

A brief discussion of the various time-restricted eating protocols as well as their respective pros and cons and implementation.

Intermittent fasting can help us achieve our goals.

Be they health-related, or simply weight loss and/or fat loss goals.

Often these are linked.

Before we dive into the nuts and bolts of intermittent fasting there is one thing that needs to be mentioned.

We must realize that intermittent fasting is a tool to be used in conjunction with an overall healthy approach to diet and nutrition.

We already know that a calorie is not just a calorie.

We know that the source of our calories matters a great deal.

This is true on a macro-nutrient level (do our calories come from protein, fats or carbohydrates?)

It is also true on a micro-nutrient level (certain foods contain certain vitamins and minerals. We need a whole bunch of different minerals and vitamins. Ergo, we need a whole bunch of different foods).

We also know that intermittent fasting can therefore not be used as a license to eat whatever crap you feel like, in whatever quantity you feel like.

You cannot out fast a crappy diet.

You also can't out train a crappy diet.

What you eat still matters just as much when you do intermittent fasting as it does when consuming food throughout the day.

Cool. Let's move on.

A calorie might not be a calorie, but reducing daily calories will still result in weight loss.

Fasting makes it easier to achieve the desired caloric restriction.

Because you can eat fewer normal sized meals during an intermittent fasting protocol.

As opposed to many (6-8) small, unfulfilling meals as required by various diets.

One or two regular meals is psychologically far easier, and for most of us more natural, that having a bunch of small, non-satisfying meals throughout the day.

Not to mention the improved logistics of not having to prep and carry around all day those "6-8 small meals" each and every damn day.

Intermittent fasting is therefore also potentially far more affordable. Obviously depending on what exactly you buy to eat.

Intermittent fasting is infinitely easier to maintain than preparing and carrying all those small meals every day.

In fact, the improved logistics of intermittent fasting may be my favorite aspect of it.

Intermittent fasting also therefore saves time.

Time not spent meal prepping and packing is time saved for doing other things.

Okay, nuts and bolts time.

We're going to discuss various forms of intermittent fasting protocols.

But is important to note that there is no one correct method of intermittent fasting.

The best method of intermittent fasting is the method that works for you.

You can also combine elements of the different fasting protocols to customize a way of eating that fits in with your lifestyle.

Factors such as what type of job you do, when you work, when you have your workouts (if indeed you have any), what type of workouts you do, etc all need to be taken account of in order for you to develop a protocol that fits your life.

The 16/8 protocol:

This means a 16 hours fasted, 8 hours eating window.

Usually, this means simply skipping breakfast.

You can then consume two larger meals throughout the day, typically lunch and dinner.

This means that a good portion of your fasting window is spent sleeping, making the whole fast easier.

Note, 16 hours is the minimum fasting time suggested.

This is because it takes a while for your body to become depleted enough to induce autophagy.

You also want to stay in the fasted state for a while in order to benefit from higher levels of human growth hormone secretion and autophagy.

So you can choose to modify the 16/8 protocol for a longer fast; i.e. an 18/6, 20/4, 22/2, etc.

It's very important that you trust the beneficial aspects of intermittent fasting.

Many people who also weight train and have as their goal an increase in muscle size are fearful of intermittent fasting.

These fears are unfounded.

But because of this, many fasters who hit the gym in the morning will take Branched Chain Amino Acids before heading out.

The theory is that the BCAA's will provide building materials for muscle growth whilst maintaining a fasted state.

I believe this to be untrue.

However, it depends on your definition of fasting.

Some proponents of intermittent fasting state that consumption of more than 50 calories constitutes breaking a fast.

Other proponents suggest that the secretion of insulin is what constitutes a broken fast.

If you agree with the first premise then, by all means, take your BCAA's.

I, however, see a fast as being broken due to the secretion of insulin.

This is because insulin causes an end to the secretion of HGH and autophagy.

If you agree with this definition then rather train in a completely fasted state.

After a period of adjustment, you will find that a fasted state does not diminish your performance in the gym.

It might take a few days for your body to become used to training on an empty stomach, but eventually, you will be able to lift just as heavy and as intensely in a fasted state as you did during your previous fed workouts.

It is also not worth freaking out after your workouts with regards to eating.

You will not waste away and forego your gains if you don't eat the second you walk out of the gym.

Your body is smarter than you think.

In fact, it may be useful to wait an hour or two to eat after your workout.

This is because you will benefit from the elevated levels of human growth hormone that a fasted state provides.

You will also have increased insulin sensitivity and glycogen depletion.

Therefore your body will be primed to eat.

Meaning that when you do eat your body will use the food to grow and store in your muscles.

In this way, you can achieve the holy grail of body recomposition.

You can lose fat AND grow muscle at the same time.

So, if you train in the morning you can remain in a fasted state until lunch time.

You can have your first meal at 11:00 and your last meal at 19:00 for example.

Or 10:00 and 18:00.

Or 12:00 and 20:00.

Or you can shorten the eating window to perhaps a 20/4 protocol and have your first meal at 12:00 and your last meal at 16:00 for example.

You can adjust in an infinite number of ways.

As long as your protocol allows a 16-hour minimum fasted state and fits in with your lifestyle.

Some people even skip dinner instead of breakfast.

They might hit the gym in the morning, eat breakfast afterward and then lunch a couple of hours after breakfast, hitting the gym in a deeply fasted state the following day again.

You can workout during the day, during the evening or during the morning.

You can have a short amount of time fasted before your workout followed by a longer time fasted after your workout.

You can have a longer fasted period (perhaps even overnight) before your workout and a smaller amount of fasted time (even immediately following a workout) time after a workout.

Your body is more adaptable and intelligent than you think.

You will not lose muscle mass (keep those gains bro!) or enter into a famine state where your metabolism slows down.

Don't overthink things.

Simply train when you like to.

Simply eat when it suits you.

Keep things simple.

Other protocols:

OMAD - One Meal A Day.

The OMAD protocol is my personal favorite.

It works because I simply skip eating during the day and then I enjoy a delicious meal at night.

No meal prep or going out for lunch.

No carrying around little plastic containers of food.

Just simplicity and freedom.

The same rules as the 16/8 protocol apply.

Only now you consume one meal per day.

One meal effectively means an eating window of approximately an hour.

So you may enjoy a nice big plate of food and perhaps even some "seconds" or even a healthy dessert such as some prebiotic yogurt with berries, honey, and fruit.

Of course, the exact foods you consume, based on the diet you choose to follow, will predetermine this.

Also worth noting is that fasted means FASTED.

No calories are consumed during the day.

This means only black, sugar-free coffee or tea and/or water during the day.

And skip the sweeteners, as most of them will still trigger an insulin response even if they don't contain any calories.

Also, most sweeteners are poison.

You don't need them.

This protocol seems restrictive. Indeed it is. But I find it freeing. I don't need to concern myself with food and drink during the day.

This means I can get on with doing other things.

It's efficient.

However, it may not work for you.

Remember, the best intermittent fasting protocol is the one that works for you.

I often train in the morning and then only eat at night.

I haven't lost muscle mass.

I haven't died, contrary to what most gym bros will have you believe.

Try it and see for yourself.

The Alternate Day Protocol:

This is where you would eat 3 regular meals during the first day, then forgo food the next day (essentially a 24 hour fast) and then eat normally again the on the third day.

For example:

Monday - Breakfast 08:00, lunch 12:00, dinner 19:00

Tuesday - Nothing. Nada. No food until 19:00. Then one meal.

Wednesday - Breakfast 08:00, lunch 12:00, dinner 19:00

Thursday - Nothing until 19:00. Then only one meal, etc..

You don't need to have the 24 hour fast every second day either.

Try once per week, or twice per week, or whatever works for you.

You can also throw in a 24 fast into one of the other protocols every now and then.

Just to switch things up a bit.

Go ahead. Just try it.

Chapter 8 - Clarifications.

A chapter on how long you need to fast, what you may consume during a fast, what to eat when breaking a fast and what to eat for the greatest health and disease-fighting benefits.

So, let's use this chapter to tie everything we've learned into a neat little bow.

Eating is important.

We need food for all of the functions our bodies are continuously engaged in.

What we eat matters a great deal.

A calorie is not simply a calorie.

For cancer-fighting a low carbohydrate way of eating is preferable.

A fast needs to last for at least 16 hours.

This is important as it allows your body time to engage in autophagy.

For optimal results don't consume any calories during a fast.

This means only black, unsweetened coffee or tea or water.

Skip the sweeteners.

If you eat a heavy meal with starchy carbs (such as potatoes for example), grains and/or legumes (beans and lentils as an example) and meat then try to first consume something lighter before.

This means that you could consume bone broth or a salad or some kefir about a half an hour before your main meal.

This basically just preps the digestive system.

It tells the digestive system "okay, we're getting some food, prepare the stomach and intestines".

This isn't strictly necessary, however consuming a heavy meal on an empty stomach can make you feel very full, tired and possibly bloated.

A healthy green juice or smoothie is another great meal to prepare the stomach for the larger meal later on.

You can have workouts as normal whilst following an intermittent fasting protocol.

You will have enough stored glycogen in your muscles for your body to use as fuel.

You won't lose your gains if you don't eat directly after a workout.

Being in a prolonged fasted state will also allow your body to use the food you ingest as muscle fuel first.

Your depleted glycogen stores will be filled up first.

This means less food (if any) being stored as fat.

Double win.

Fasting coupled with decent sleep also leads to higher amounts of human growth hormone secretion.

This alone will help you drop body fat whilst increasing those gains.

The moderate amount of stress fasting entails boosts your body's disease-fighting capabilities, including its cancer-fighting abilities.

Listen to your body.

Especially if you train regularly.

If you feel weak and "off" check to see if you are consuming enough water.

Are you sleeping well?

Are you eating enough protein and carbs during your eating window?

If yes to all the above then don't worry about going off of your intermittent fasting protocol for a few days.

Simply get back on the horse when you feel capable of it.

Learn to listen to your body.

Don't overthink and overanalyze intermittent fasting.

Don't aim for perfection.

Aim for consistency over the long term.

If you're starting out and a 16/8 fast (or longer) seems too difficult then start out with what you are capable of.

If you can only fast for 14 hours, then good! Build from there.

Aim to have a significant amount of time fasted as part of sleep.

It's easy to not think of food when you're sleeping.

For women, abstain from fasting when you are pregnant.

If you are experiencing a period of increased stress (massive project and short deadlines at work for example) and you start to feel fatigued then consider not fasting for a few days.

Fasting does induce stress. It's the good type of stress though. But you don't want to add stress to your body when severely taxed.

This is true for men and women.

But don't go off the rails completely. Eating garbage places much more stress on your body than skipping a few meals.

Afterword:

To the reader

It has been a great pleasure to research and write this book.

As a practitioner of intermittent fasting that has seen and felt the amazing difference it makes

I knew that there was something to intermittent fasting.

The current hype is not overblown.

Writing this book was amazing for me as I came to know some of the science behind intermittent fasting.

Needless to say, I find it fascinating.

My hope for you is that this book has helped explain in easy terms to you what intermittent fasting is all about.

The book also attempts to show the various metabolic and physiological benefits that intermittent fasting holds.

It aims to explain these in easy to understand terminology.

I also wanted to discuss how to do intermittent fasting as well as what foods should be consumed during the eating window.

My sincerest hope is that I delivered at least some of the above to you.

I want the whole world to feel and experience first hand the dramatic difference intermittent fasting can have in our lives.

More energy, more time, less fatigue, fewer illnesses and a potentially deadly weapon against cancer.

But don't worry too much about the science.

A lot of it is still being discovered and expanded on.

Simply try intermittent fasting yourself and see if it works for you.

Chances are that it will change your life.

In fact, I am confident of it.

Thank you for purchasing this book.

Your support is deeply appreciated.

Wishing you robust health and true happiness.

Many Thanks.
Lawrence

Resources: Other books by J. Lawrence Tine

KILL YOUR DISEASE

USING THE SCIENCE BEHIND CELLULAR RENEWAL AND AUTOPHAGY TO KILL YOUR DISEASES AND BUILD A BRAND NEW YOU.

Revealed in an easy-to-understand way is the ONE THING that everyone can do, right now, in order to dramatically improve overall health.

One powerful thing that almost all people can do right now to:

- Improve your overall markers for health, leading to a significantly healthier YOU.
- Reverse the effects of aging. A younger you, explained by easy-to-understand science.
- Kill the bad cells in your body (causing you harm and a host of health problems) whilst preserving and rebuilding the healthy cells your body needs.

- Rebuilding your body at the cellular level. Re-creating your body to function in an optimal way.
- Resetting the immune system leading to lower levels of inflammation and a significant decrease in auto-immune issues.
- Lower levels of insulin and reduce the harmful effects that increased insulin levels have on your body.
- Increase insulin response and insulin sensitivity.
- Enjoy optimal digestion.

In this 8 part book, we look at exactly where your health may have gone wrong.

Hint: It's not that you haven't found the right medication yet.

Many times diseases are overlooked by well-meaning doctors that focus on symptoms instead of origins.

If we can discover the origin of an ailment then we can also discover potential cures.

Identifying and managing symptoms only causes you long term poor health outcomes.

So it pays to know what's going on in your body.

In this book you'll discover:

- The 1 powerful secret that many professionals overlook when discussing issues of health.

- The one simple thing you can do to reverse many of the signs and drawbacks of aging

- The one (very important) thing you can do, right now, to reverse many modern diseases.

- Why stress (the right kind) is beneficial and even crucial to optimal health.

- How to get rid of sub-optimal cells in your body, and replace them by brand new, optimal cells.

- How "eating yourself" may end up saving your life.

So even if you don't know anything about cellular renewal, this comprehensive guide will put you on the right path.

KILL YOUR DISEASE By J. Lawrence Tine. SEARCH FOR IT ON AMAZON TODAY!

Other books by Archboard Publishing:

Affirmations: The no-nonsense book on the power and purpose of affirmations.

By James L. Corsair

Amazon ASIN: B01MUBE48F

One man's journey in learning how to become stress free, form new habits, reject negative thoughts, live in the moment and become much happier in the process!

A no-nonsense book on Affirmations: The way they work and what they can do for you!

Book Description.

Greetings Friend,

My name is James Corsair and I am the author of

"The no-nonsense book on the power and purpose of affirmations".

This book is about the power and reality of affirmations and how you can use them to lead a better, healthier, less stressed-out life. From skeptic to believer, including the system that aided my transformation from stressed out, self sabotaging, negative person into a calm, controlled and much MUCH happier person - It's all in here.

Inside this book I show you the secret to using affirmations in order to interrupt negative and self-destructive thoughts and behaviors and the step-by-step process that will empower you to analyze your own stumbling blocks and design your own affirmations to combat your own negative thoughts and self destructive behavior.

Start using Affirmations today and experience amazing, life changing benefits.

- Are you constantly sabotaging your own progress?
- Do you wish to understand why you do the things you do?
- Would you like to be able to rewire your responses and behavior?
- Do you wish to rediscover your discipline, willpower and become the person that you were meant to be?

Affirmations can help you learn new ways of thinking to stop you from sabotaging your own growth and potential.

Learn to use affirmations today.

Become the "you" that you always knew you could be!

Affirmations have the potential to transform your entire life! The information in this book has as its aim exactly that: To aid you, the reader, in finally quitting bad behavior and negative thinking, and finally start doing the things that you know you should be doing.

Affirmations have the ability to change your entire life!

You are about to discover how to:

- Become aware of your negative thought patterns and emotional responses
- Let go of the hurt, anger and regret holding you back
- Become actively aware of your mental and emotional state
- Reject negative thoughts and emotions
- Interrupt and rewire your old ways of thinking
- Reduce stress and anxiety
- Achieve the emotional and mental state that is the truest you
- Set the stage emotionally for massive growth and reaching your fullest potential
- And much, much more!

Download your copy today!
Take action today and download this book.
Amazon ASIN: B01MUBE48F

Positive Thinking: 8 Simple steps to achieving SUCCESS, HAPPINESS and finally reaching your GOALS!

By James L. Corsair
Amazon ASIN: B01MS8DN9C

Positive Thinking: 8 Simple steps to achieving SUCCESS, HAPPINESS and finally reaching your GOALS

Download your copy today!

Amazon ASIN: B01MS8DN9C

Mindfulness: The Mindfulness Experiment. A no-nonsense book on mindfulness - One man's journey in learning how to chill out, be happy and live in the moment!

By James L. Corsair
Amazon ASIN: B01MU8NJGJ

One man's journey in learning how to chill out, be happy and live in the moment! A no-nonsense book on mindfulness

Book Description.

Hello there, Dear Friend

My name is James Corsair and am the author of

"The Mindfulness Experiment".

This book chronicles my journey from skeptic to believer, as well as my transformation from being a stressed out, burned out, nervous breakdown suffering victim into a happy, positive and calm victor.

And Inside this book I reveal to you my secret to building a foundation to practice Mindfulness and the proven, step-by-step process that will empower you to start practicing Mindfulness and experiencing it's amazing, powerful benefits.

- Are you stressed out and anxiety ridden?
- Do you feel directionless, aimless and purposeless?
- Are you tired and worn out?
- Do you long for calm, serenity, peace and tranquility?
- Do you wish to rediscover your old-self, become motivated to pursue your dreams, goals and ambitions and finally become the person that you know you can be?

Mindfulness can help you achieve a stress-free state and is a key part of the strategy to achieve your utmost potential. Learn to bury the memories of yesterday keeping you back and learn how to become Mindful in your day-to-day life in order to reap the benefits of a positive state and enhanced mental and emotional toughness and focus.

Become the "you" that you always knew you should be!

Mindfulness has personally transformed my entire life, The information in this book chronicles the true story, steps and strategies of my Mindfulness journey and the amazing change I've experienced as a result.

Download your copy today!

Take action today and download this book today!

Amazon ASIN: B01MU8NJGJ

References:

This book attempts to keep the science easy to understand.

I've tried to keep the book easy to read and have the information flow in a linear fashion.

However, please see the studies and references below.

It contains a ton of research and findings expounding on the information captured within this book.

I've included the below in this book for two reasons:

Firstly as reference and acknowledgement of the work that has been done by minds far greater than mine.

Secondly, as an additional resource for you to use in order to facilitate further study.

I hope you find it useful and stimulating.

Enjoy.

Levine I. Cancer among the American Indians and its bearing upon the ethnological distribution of the disease. J Cancer Res Clin Oncol. 1910;9:422–435.

Orenstein AJ. Freedom Of Negro Races From Cancer. Br Med J. 1923;2:342.

Prentice G. Cancer Among Negroes. Br Med J. 1923;2:1181.

Brown GM, Cronk LB, Boag TJ. The occurrence of cancer in an Eskimo. Cancer. 1952;5:142–143. 10.1002/1097-0142(195201)5:1<142::AID-CNCR2820050119>3.0.CO;2-Q.

Eaton SB, Konner M, Shostak M. Stone agers in the fast lane: chronic degenerative diseases in evolutionary perspective. Am J Med. 1988;84:739–749. doi: 10.1016/0002-9343(88)90113-1.

Carrera-Bastos P, Fontes-Villalba M, O'Keefe JH, Lindeberg S, Cordain L. The western diet and lifestyle and diseases of civilization. Research Reports in Clinical Cardiology. 2011;2:15–35.

Weinberg SL. The diet-heart hypothesis: a critique. J Am Coll Cardiol. 2004;43:731–733. 10.1016/j.jacc.2003.10.034.

Henderson ST. High carbohydrate diets and Alzheimer's disease. Med Hypotheses. 2004;62:689–700. 1016/j.mehy.2003.11.028.

Seneff S, Wainwright G, Mascitelli L. Nutrition and Alzheimer's disease: the detrimental role of a high carbohydrate diet. Eur J Intern Med. 2011;22:134–140. 10.1016/j.ejim.2010.12.017.

Chiu CJ, Milton RC, Gensler G, Taylor A. Dietary carbohydrate intake and glycemic index in relation to cortical and nuclear lens opacities in the Age-Related Eye Disease Study. Am J Clin Nutr. 2006;83:1177–1184.

Chiu CJ, Hubbard LD, Armstrong J, Rogers G, Jacques PF, Chylack LT Jr, Hankinson SE, Willett WC, Taylor A. Dietary glycemic index and carbohydrate in relation to early age-related macular degeneration. Am J Clin Nutr. 2006;83:880–886.

Kaushik S, Wang JJ, Flood V, Tan JS, Barclay AW, Wong TY, Brand-Miller J, Mitchell P. Dietary glycemic index and the risk of age-related macular degeneration. Am J Clin Nutr. 2008;88:1104–1110.

Dessein PH, Shipton EA, Stanwix AE, Joffe BI, Ramokgadi J. Beneficial effects of weight loss associated with moderate calorie/carbohydrate restriction, and increased proportional intake of protein and unsaturated fat on serum urate and lipoprotein levels in gout: a pilot study. Ann Rheum Dis. 2000;59:539–543. 10.1136/ard.59.7.539.

Roe CM, Fitzpatrick AL, Xiong C, Sieh W, Kuller L, Miller JP, Williams MM, Kopan R, Behrens MI, Morris JC. Cancer linked to Alzheimer disease but not vascular dementia. Neurology. 2010;74:106–112. 10.1212/WNL.0b013e3181c91873.

Boffetta P, Nordenvall C, Nyren O, Ye W. A prospective study of gout and cancer. Eur J Cancer Prev. 2009;18:127–132. 10.1097/CEJ.0b013e328313631a.

Braun S, Bitton-Worms K, Leroith D. The Link between the Metabolic Syndrome and Cancer. Int J Biol Sci. 2011;7:1003–1015.

Cheung N, Shankar A, Klein R, Folsom AR, Couper DJ, Wong TY. Age-related macular degeneration and cancer mortality in the atherosclerosis risk in communities study. Arch Ophthalmol. 2007;125:1241–1247. 10.1001/archopht.125.9.1241.

Derr RL, Ye X, Islas MU, Desideri S, Saudek CD, Grossman SA. Association between hyperglycemia and survival in patients with newly diagnosed glioblastoma. J Clin Oncol. 2009;27:1082–1086. 10.1200/JCO.2008.19.1098.

Goodwin PJ, Ennis M, Pritchard KI, Trudeau ME, Koo J, Madarnas Y, Hartwick W, Hoffman B, Hood N. Fasting insulin and outcome in early-stage breast cancer: results of a prospective cohort study. J Clin Oncol. 2002;20:42–51. 10.1200/JCO.20.1.42.

Ma J, Li H, Giovannucci E, Mucci L, Qiu W, Nguyen PL, Gaziano JM, Pollak M, Stampfer MJ. Prediagnostic body-mass index, plasma C-peptide concentration, and prostate cancer-specific mortality in men with prostate cancer: a long-term survival analysis. Lancet Oncol. 2008;9:1039–1047. 10.1016/S1470-2045(08)70235-3.

Stattin P, Bjor O, Ferrari P, Lukanova A, Lenner P, Lindahl B, Hallmans G, Kaaks R. Prospective study of hyperglycemia and cancer risk. Diabetes Care. 2007;30:561–567. 10.2337/dc06-0922.

Weiser MA, Cabanillas ME, Konopleva M, Thomas DA, Pierce SA, Escalante CP, Kantarjian HM, O'Brien SM. Relation between the duration of remission and hyperglycemia during induction chemotherapy for acute lymphocytic leukemia with a hyperfractionated cyclophosphamide, vincristine, doxorubicin, and dexamethasone/methotrexate-cytarabine regimen. Cancer. 2004;100:1179–1185. 10.1002/cncr.20071.

Wolpin BM, Meyerhardt JA, Chan AT, Ng K, Chan JA, Wu K, Pollak MN, Giovannucci EL, Fuchs CS. Insulin, the insulin-like growth factor axis, and mortality in patients with nonmetastatic colorectal cancer. J Clin Oncol. 2009;27:176–185. 10.1200/JCO.2008.17.9945.

Yuhara H, Steinmaus C, Cohen SE, Corley DA, Tei Y, Buffler PA. Is Diabetes Mellitus an Independent Risk Factor for Colon Cancer and Rectal Cancer? Am J Gastroenterol.2011.

Augustin LS, Dal Maso L, La Vecchia C, Parpinel M, Negri E, Vaccarella S, Kendall CW, Jenkins DJ, Francesch S. Dietary glycemic index and glycemic load, and breast cancer risk: a case-control study. Ann Oncol. 2001;12:1533–1538. 10.1023/A:1013176129380.

Melnik BC, John SM, Schmitz G. Over-stimulation of insulin/IGF1 signaling by Western diet may promote diseases of civilization: lessons learnt from Laron syndrome. Nutr Metab (Lond) 2011;8:41. 10.1186/1743-7075-8-41.

Sieri S, Pala V, Brighenti F, Pellegrini N, Muti P, Micheli A, Evangelista A, Grioni S, Contiero P, Berrino F, Krogh V. Dietary glycemic index, glycemic load, and the risk of breast cancer in an Italian prospective cohort study. Am J Clin Nutr. 2007;86:1160–1166.

32Wen W, Shu XO, Li H, Yang G, Ji BT, Cai H, Gao YT, Zheng W. Dietary carbohydrates, fiber, and breast cancer risk in Chinese women. Am J Clin Nutr. 2009;89:283–289.

Warburg O. Über den Stoffwechsel der Carzinomzelle. Klinische Wochenschrift. 1925. pp. 534–536.

Warburg O, Posener K, Negelein E. Über den Stoffwechsel der Carcinomzelle. Biochem Zeitschr. 1924. pp. 309–344.

Warburg O, Wind F, Negelein E. Über den Stoffwechsel der Tumoren im Körper. Klinische Wochenschrift. 1926. pp. 828–832.

Koppenol WH, Bounds PL, Dang CV. Otto Warburg's contributions to current concepts of cancer metabolism. Nat Rev Cancer. 2011;11:325–337. 10.1038/nrc3038.

Demetrakopoulos GE, Linn B, Amos H. Rapid loss of ATP by tumor cells deprived of glucose: contrast to normal cells. Biochem Biophys Res Commun. 1978;82:787–794. 10.1016/0006-291X(78)90851-3.

Priebe A, Tan L, Wahl H, Kueck A, He G, Kwok R, Opipari A, Liu JR. Glucose deprivation activates AMPK and induces cell death through modulation of Akt in ovarian cancer cells. Gynecol Oncol. 2011;122:389–95. 10.1016/j.ygyno.2011.04.024.

Shim H, Chun YS, Lewis BC, Dang CV. A unique glucose-dependent apoptotic pathway induced by c-Myc. Proc Natl Acad Sci USA. 1998;95:1511–1516. 10.1073/pnas.95.4.1511.

Masur K, Vetter C, Hinz A, Tomas N, Henrich H, Niggemann B, Zanker KS. Diabetogenic glucose and insulin concentrations modulate transcriptome and protein levels involved in tumour cell migration, adhesion and proliferation. Br J Cancer. 2011;104:345–352. 10.1038/sj.bjc.6606050.

Santisteban GA, Ely JT, Hamel EE, Read DH, Kozawa SM. Glycemic modulation of tumor tolerance in a mouse model of breast cancer. Biochem Biophys Res Commun. 1985;132:1174–1179. 10.1016/0006-291X(85)91930-8.

Seyfried TN, Sanderson TM, El-Abbadi MM, McGowan R, Mukherjee P. Role of glucose and ketone bodies in the metabolic control of experimental brain cancer. Br J Cancer. 2003;89:1375–1382. 10.1038/sj.bjc.6601269.

Shanmugam N, Reddy MA, Guha M, Natarajan R. High glucose-induced expression of proinflammatory cytokine and chemokine genes in monocytic cells. Diabetes. 2003;52:1256–1264. 10.2337/diabetes.52.5.1256.

Wen Y, Gu J, Li SL, Reddy MA, Natarajan R, Nadler JL. Elevated glucose and diabetes promote interleukin-12 cytokine gene expression in mouse macrophages. Endocrinology. 2006;147:2518–2525. 10.1210/en.2005-0519.

Dandona P, Chaudhuri A, Ghanim H, Mohanty P. Proinflammatory effects of glucose and anti-inflammatory effect of insulin: relevance to cardiovascular disease. Am J Cardiol. 2007;99:15B–26B.

Pollak M. Insulin and insulin-like growth factor signalling in neoplasia. Nat Rev Cancer. 2008;8:915–928. 10.1038/nrc2536.

Händel M, Tadeuma K. Über die Beziehung des Geschwulstwachstums zur Ernährung und zum Stoffwechsel. II. Mitteilung. Versuche zur Frage der Bedeutung der Kohlenhydrate für das Wachstum des Rattencarcinoms. Klin Wochenschr. 1924. pp. 288–293.

Seyfried TN, Shelton LM. Cancer as a metabolic disease. Nutr Metab (Lond) 2010;7:7. 10.1186/1743-7075-7-7.

https://www.ncbi.nlm.nih.gov/pmc/articles/PMC3267662/ Is there a role for carbohydrate restriction in the treatment and prevention of cancer? Rainer J Klement and Ulrike Kämmerer.

National Center for Biotechnology Information

PubMed Central® (PMC) is a free full-text archive of biomedical and life sciences journal literature at the U.S. National Institutes of Health's National Library of Medicine (NIH/NLM).

US National Library of Medicine

US National Institutes of Health